Disaster Survival

How To Survive a Disaster

The practical Guide (Tornado, Hurricane,

Earthquake, Avalanche, and More)

Table of Contents

INTRODUCTION

Congratulations on downloading this book and thank you for doing so.

We live in tumultuous times. Every day we wake up completely unaware of the threats that are surrounding us. Aside from having to be on guard from the natural elements of a disaster we also have to concern ourselves with the human factor. This means that each of us has to keep foremost in our minds escape plans, extra stores of food, and other tools we may need to protect our families and property at all times.

In the past, when a disaster occurred, it was most likely a surprise. People woke because their houses are flooded, properties uprooted from violent shaking from earthquakes, volcanoes erupted suffocating people with their intense heat and gases, and the sea floor rose claiming millions of lives without warning. All these types of events left behind millions of people in their wake stunned and grieved over their losses.

Even today, you turn on the latest news reports and see almost daily about earthquakes, floods, fires, typhoons, tornadoes, and so many more natural disasters. To some, it may feel like the earth is angry and bent on destroying anyone in its path. The expression, "you can't fight mother nature," seems to be on the lips of the whole world.

The good news though is that we are now living in a technologically advanced time. While we can't accurately predict the future, man has developed a means of understanding nature and how it works. As a result, when these things do occur, we now have the foresight to see them coming giving us a chance to prepare. No longer do disasters have to take so many lives. People are now more aware of the types of natural events that may affect their area and can do something about it.

According to a report from the World Bank, right now, more than 160 countries have a large part of their population that is considered to be living in high mortality zones from exposure to natural disasters. And many scientists are now pointing out that humans are actually putting more people in harm's way by encouraging massive populations to live in such danger zones.

So, even if the disaster itself turns out to not be life-threatening, other factors can escalate the situations. Unplanned urbanization, the deforestation of large regions of land, and the extensive amount of manmade products (like concrete, metal structures, and asphalt) disrupt the natural flow of water and prevent the earth from proper draining has created other hazards that can compound the risks of a true natural event.

Add to that human frustration on a political, religious, and economic level, which creates a whole new type of disaster that we must contend with. We now have to deal with human frustration as it presents itself in the form of terrorist attacks, public shootings, and other forms of violence where people have become so overwhelmed they fight back. Yes, if there was ever a time for specialized training in disaster preparedness it is now.

In this book, we will discuss fundamental lessons that we all must learn to prepare for the inevitability that one day we will be faced with one of these disasters. We all need to:

- Learn to recognize the warning signs

- Develop basic principles that can help us to save lives

- Be proactive and know what to do before an event happens

- Find out what types of disaster are a high risk for your area

- And how to keep safe in the chaos left in the wake of a disaster

In the following chapters, we will teach you how to protect yourself when help is not available and what to do before, during, and after a catastrophic event to ensure the safety of those you care for.

No one looks forward to these types of surprises, but we all know that one day a tragic event will befall most of us. Being forewarned is to be forearmed. It is time for all of us to be more conscious about our environment and our surroundings so that we can be prepared for the next time disaster strikes.

There are plenty of books on this subject on the market, thanks again for choosing this one! Every effort was made to ensure it is full of as much useful information as possible, please enjoy!

CHAPTER 1

AN INTRODUCTION TO DISASTER SURVIVAL

At the end of 2017, CNBC, a major news channel made a profound observation. They declared that 2017 as one of the most devastating years for disasters. Reports of catastrophic floods, earthquakes, hurricanes, and wildfires spread around the globe at an alarming rate. Global insurance companies lost billions of dollars and faced the third-most expensive year in their industry.

The fact is, today no one is immune from disaster. It is the one type of event that can affect us all regardless of economic status, where we live, or ethnic background. We read about these events almost on a daily basis, and it sends chills down our spine. But it is one thing to hear about the tragedy that has befallen someone and shake our heads in sadness at the poor unfortunate people, and it is another thing to be ripped from sleep as our whole world shatters around us.

Our only protection from such events is to prepare ahead of time and know exactly what to do when one of these tragic events actually happens to us. But while most of us are fully aware of the threats that loom over us every day, few of us know exactly what to do when it happens. Preparing for a disaster is not just about gathering things together for our physical protection, but one must also have some mental preparation as well. Without psychologically recognizing the threat, it is hard to seriously follow through with the physical work one needs to do to protect their family.

Psychological Preparation

It is difficult for many of us to imagine our lives being turned upside down by some unexpected disaster. We have been told for years about the risks in our area, and still many refuse to recognize the potential danger they may be living in every day. One of the first steps needed to prepare for a disaster mentally is to acknowledge that the threats are real.

Every day people are content to ignore the warning signs in hopes that the threats that loom over us will not really materialize but we've seen time and time again that when it comes to disasters, it is not a question of "if" a major event will take place but "when." By acknowledging that disasters can and will happen, you can mentally prepare yourself for their inevitability. These steps must be done beforehand because in most cases, preparation after the fact is rarely possible. You want to be proactive when something happens, not reactive.

Things get much easier once you've taken this step. Once your mind has accepted the fact that disasters will continue to happen no matter where we live, you can start to prepare yourself for what is to come. While the same disasters do not happen in the same way all over the globe, the reality is that your area is subject to some kind of disaster and you need to know what it is.

In America, every section of the country is divided up into disaster zones. California is susceptible to major earthquakes, wildfires, and record heat. Florida and parts of the east coast are susceptible to hurricanes and flooding. Areas surrounding large bodies of water are at risk of flooding, and coastal areas are always at risk of a potential tsunami triggered by an event that may have occurred thousands of miles away.

The more you learn about the disasters that your area is at high risk of experiencing, the easier it will be for you to take the necessary steps to prepare yourself for what will one day come.

It is important to understand that preparation itself does not guarantee that you will not be affected by these events, but it certainly does give you a better chance. A forest fire ripping through your neighborhood may not spare your home but preparation could spare your life and that of your family. At the very least, you should know where the shelters are, reinforce your home to withstand the pressures it may face, and eliminate the hazards that could cause harm and injury to those inside. But all of these things start with the psychological preparation for a disaster.

What effective preparation can do is take away much of the fear, anxiety, and reduce a great deal of the tragic losses that disasters bring. It lays the groundwork for those in your immediate family and community to know what to do if something were to happen.

As the saying goes, "knowledge is power." Being ready to evacuate, knowing where to seek refuge, and how to ensure that your basic needs are met are the key to survival in this unpredictable world.

Every year, hundreds of thousands of lives are lost because of a lack of preparation. A disastrous event may last only a few seconds, but its impact on people and property could linger for years. The assumption that the government will readily swoop in and rescue you is a major misnomer. Yes FEMA is there, local police are available, and fire service/paramedics are on call and are just a few buttons away. But, when millions in a single area are affected, their services may be hours, if not days, away. In fact, they may, and most likely will, be suffering and trying to recover from the same disaster. You must be mentally prepared for the fact that they may not be able to get to you or that there are others who need more help than you do.

It is up to you to know how to respond to any disastrous situation that may occur in your area, no matter what it may be. At the very least, this should involve making sure you have food, shelter, clothing, water, sanitation, and first aid. If you have all these things already prepared, waiting for help will be a lot easier and definitely less stressful.

The Difference Between Being Proactive and Reactive

Everywhere, when catastrophic events strike people will be either proactive or reactive, so it pays to understand the difference between these two. Both will get you to the end of your journey, but the kind of journey you take will depend largely on which route you take.

Proactive people plan ahead for a crucial disaster whereas reactive people are more inclined to think on the fly. When you are proactive, you are thinking about the people you care for, the structure you have to protect, any equipment or supplies you will need, and planning to reduce any exposure to risk that you may have to undergo.

If you are reactive, you will only react to an event after it happens (or just before it happens if you get a warning). If news of a hurricane is approaching, you will be among the throngs of people stripping the cupboards bare in the supermarket in the days and hours before the storm hits. You'll be frantically making calls on your cell phone looking for safe haven, and you'll be the one short on fuel when the lines for gas stations stretch out for miles on end. Clearly, being reactive may get you where you want to be, but you'll be getting quite a few cuts and bruises along the way.

Of course, when you are proactive, there is no way o prepare for every eventuality, but you will at least,

- Have supplies on hand

- Have a plan of action in place so that everyone in the household knows what to do

- Have rehearsed that plan to identify its weaknesses

- Have supplies available for every person in the household

- Have considered medical conditions for everyone

- Have considered what to do to protect your pets

- And have an evacuation plan ready to execute if needed.

Disasters are extremely stressful. Every event comes with its own anxieties and challenges, but if you want to smooth out many of the rough edges you will be pushed up against, you need to be proactive. Your main goal is to protect your family as much as is humanly possible from these catastrophic events and you can only do that through being proactive. To do this, you need to develop a plan for what to do before, during, and after a disaster strikes.

CHAPTER 2

DISASTERS – WHAT EVERYONE NEEDS TO KNOW

When preparing for a major disaster one of the first things people want to do is arm themselves with knowledge about their risk exposure. Every one of us is part of a national infrastructure that is interdependent on each other for support, and that is where most will turn when something disastrous happens.

In America, we are fortunate to have such a solid infrastructure in place. Think about the many countries who are not as advanced as we are and how their people must fend for themselves if something were to happen. People end up roaming the streets for days in search of food or water, families are often forced to separate, and disease runs rampant. But, sometimes we tend to take these services for granted, assuming they will always be available when in reality, these systems may be just as vulnerable to a catastrophic event as we are. For that reason, it is more important than ever to accumulate knowledge to make sure that you are safe when something happens.

There are three periods you must be concerned with. What to do before an event strikes; this is where the majority of disaster preparedness happens. The more knowledge you have about the event, the better prepared you can be. To begin with, you need to:

- Learn as much as you can about the risks and dangers you are exposed to in your area.

- Obtain the necessary insurance in the event of destruction of life and property

- Develop plans for what to do if you need to evacuate your home

- Gather together any necessary supplies you may need

- Rehearse any plan so you can identify weaknesses or problems and make the necessary adjustments.

When a disaster does strike, you should also have knowledge of what to do when you're right in the middle of it. If you've planned well, everyone in your household will know exactly what to do, where to go, and how to survive the situation. They will be able to put their plan into action and may even be in a position to offer assistance to others who may be in need. They will also be aware of the risks they are exposed to and where to seek cover and protection when an event happens.

And after the event, they will know what steps to take to secure their safety, and even what to do to prevent harm to life and property after the fact. All of this sounds simple enough, but none of it is possible without proper planning. There are some basic things that everyone, regardless of the type of disaster they may be facing can do to prepare for what is to come.

Basic Needs Everyone Should Have on Hand

As you start creating your disaster plan, you need to think about the unique needs of your household. It helps to get everyone together so that you can have an open and frank conversation about what you can realistically expect to accomplish to meet your daily needs.

While you may be able to expect governmentally support, it is very important that you create your own network of people, each with his or her own responsibilities already in place. Things you can discuss in this meeting:

- The differing ages of those in your household and what responsibilities you can expect each one to perform successfully

- The locations each of you may be in when a disaster strikes

- Dietary needs

- Health and medical needs each one has

- How to care for disabilities

- How to deal with language barriers if someone does not speak the local language

- What to do with your pets

- What to do if a disaster strikes and you're all separated from each other

It is important to think of your personal network as the first tier of survival preparedness. The second tier could be your outside community, workplace, school, neighbors, etc. and the third tier of protection could then rely on the government. In the moments immediately following a disaster, the first tier of your plan may be all you have to rely on.

Right after a disaster, there are a lot of things you can do to protect yourself. However, meeting your immediate needs is essential. After most disasters, power, water service, communication, and transportation in your community are most likely going to be off the grid. So, having some type of plan to compensate for these needs is crucial.

To take care of your basic needs, you may need to find an alternative means of keeping food cold, so it doesn't go bad, getting fresh water for everyone, and communicating with each other if you're separated. At the very least you need to have enough fuel in your car to evacuate, and enough food and water for each person in the household to survive, and an emergency kit stashed somewhere within easy reach. For that, you need to have a Bug Out Bag containing everything to sustain you for at least a few days.

The Bug Out Bag – What Goes in it?

The needs of your family will differ from the needs of someone else's family, but at the very least, everyone's Bug Out Bag should contain these basics:

- A change of clothes – These should be switched out with the seasons, so you are prepared for whatever season you're in. Obviously, winter clothes will not be suitable for the heat of summer, and the lighter clothes you need in the summer wouldn't be sufficient winter protection if you have to live without power for a few days.

- Sturdy shoes – Disasters leave all sorts of debris and contaminants in damaged areas. For your protection, make sure your shoes are closed in and sturdy enough to protect them from rough terrain or walking across distances that can have many unknown hazards.

- Blankets – Even in the summertime nights can be cold and unforgiving. Having blankets to protect you from the environment is essential.

- Flashlight – power will likely be off so when night falls you'll need the light to see through the darkness and flashlights could be a valuable protection from other dangers like animals and other threats that only come out at night. Make sure you have enough dry batteries to keep it working when you need it.

- Radio or some other form of portable communication – With power out, battery-operated radios could be the only connection you have to help when you need it. Because batteries stored for a long time will often fail, many also make sure they have a wind-up radio on hand. With human-generated power, you won't need to worry about keeping up to date on potential risk areas you may have to travel through. You will have continuous access to warnings about dangers and other threats that may also be coming.

- First-aid kit – These are essential to care for immediate medical needs. Injuries can be treated on the spot without the need of rushing to crowded emergency rooms whenever possible. Treatments for burns, sprains, and cuts and scratches can be attended to with the right equipment leaving those emergency facilities free to treat more severe injuries. Your first-aid kit should already be stocked with any prescription medications, and other medical supplies your family normally needs. For example, having a supply of insulin on hand for a diabetic, or inhalers for those with asthma could literally save a life.

- A whistle – If the disaster puts you in a location where you cannot extricate yourself, or you're unable to get to the help you need, having a whistle on hand to alert those outside your location where to find you.

- In addition to food, make sure you have a supply of eating utensils on hand. Canned food can last a lot longer than any other type of preserved food you may wish to store but what good is it if you haven't thought enough to pack a can opener. It helps to have a pocket tool set complete with all the utensils and supplies you need to prepare your meals. Since gas and electric may be unavailable for a time, you may need to build a fire to heat up your food so stashing some waterproof matches will also be beneficial.

- Dust masks – After major disasters, the air is often filled with dust and other irritants that could affect breathing. Having a dustproof mask to at least filter some of those particles you breathe in could help to prevent infections to lungs if you're exposed.

- Plastic sheeting or tarps – These can be used to provide temporary shelter from the elements. Plastic sheeting can be laid out on the ground or propped up and sealed with waterproof tape to keep rain and water out making it an excellent option for emergency shelter.

- Sanitary supplies – You can protect your health by keeping your hygiene up after a disaster. Make sure you have enough soap, towels, toilet paper, toothbrushes and potable water to fend off infections, bacteria, and other microscopic invaders that could compromise your health after a disaster.

- A waterproof container for holding important documents – that need to be kept safe from the elements. A waterproof container to hold your passport, driver's license, birth certificates, copies of prescriptions, insurance papers, and any other papers can save you a lot of time and grief.

- List of emergency contacts from out of the area – once news of the disaster breaks, concerned family and friends will be worried about you. A list of contacts out of the area could also give you a place to go that puts you out of immediate danger. Your list should also include a number of emergency contacts in the immediate area who could give you help when you need it.

- Credit cards and cash – banks will most likely be offline for at least a few days after a disaster. Having extra cash on hand could help you to get the things you need without having to do without.

- Extra set of house and car keys – Things can get lost easily after a disaster. Having an extra set of keys for areas you need access to will save you time from having to search through debris to find them.

- Entertainment package – especially when you have young children, having something to keep them from getting anxious can help them to cope with disaster better. If your Bug Out Bag has games, books, puzzles or anything else that is not powered electronically available it can make the transition to this change in life much easier for them.

For a time, after a disaster, you may need to go back to the old days of having paper and pencils on hand. You may have to practice writing notes rather than sending emails etc., so having these supplies on hand can make that transition so much better.

From here, your family's needs can vary from one location to the other. You may find that you need something else to add to your bag that is not included in your list. If you have elderly, disabled, or young children in your household, you have many other things to think about and prepare for.

What Should Go in Your First-Aid Kit

Having a well-stocked first aid kit is a must even when there is no impending disaster, but it can only be of help to you if it is properly stocked. Here is a list of things everyone should have on hand:

- Antiseptic wipes (alcohol based)

- Antibacterial ointment

- Bandage adhesive or a compound tincture of some kind

- An assortment of bandages in different sizes (fabric is preferred over plastic)

- Butterfly bandages or ace bandages

- Gauze pads in different sizes

- Sterile pads (preferably the non-stick type)

- Medical tape

- Blister treatments

- Pain medications

- Insect repellent

- Antihistamines to treat allergies

- Tweezers

- Safety pins

- And a first aid guidebook

Your first-aid kit needs to be able to cover several different types of injuries so aside from the basics, you should consider having these additional supplies on hand.

- Elastic wrap or ace bandages

- Triangular cravat bandages

- Splints for broken fingers

- SAM splints

- Gauze (rolled)

- Hydrogel-based pads

- Supplies for cleaning wounds

- Topical anesthetic

- Gauze for stopping blood flow (hemostatic)

- Liquid bandages

- Oval eye patches

- To protect against infections from bacteria, stock up on these supplies:

- Hand sanitizer

- Sunblock or aloe vera gel to protect from sun exposure

- Aspirin

- Antacids

- Throat lozenges

- Eye drops

- Diarrhea tablets

- Ointments for treatment of poison ivy or poison oak

- Insect repellant

- Treatment for insect bites or stings

- Glucose or another form of treatment for hypoglycemia

- Rehydration salts

- Antifungal cream (or foot powder

- Prescription medications

- Epinephrine (for treatment of allergies)

Miscellaneous items to have on hand:

- Paramedic shears

- Razor blades

- Cotton swabs

- Thermometer

- Irrigation syringe

- Magnifying glass

- Mirror (compact)

- Medical gloves

- CPR mask

- Sewing needles with thread

- Needle nose pliers/wire cutter

- Duct tape

- Medical waste bag

- Personal locator/beacon

- Satellite phone

- Lip balm

- Sunscreen

- Water treatment chemicals

- Collapsible water sink

You may not be able to obtain all the things listed here, but the more of these things you have on hand, the easier it will be for everyone in your family to cope with any type of disaster when it arrives.

Dealing With Health Issues in a Disaster

People often do not realize the extent of damage to health disasters can cause. Mental health patients are often overlooked in the wake of a traumatic event. They will be buried in among the thousands who will be walking the streets dazed and in shock. You may not be able to easily identify anyone who is suffering from a mental health disorder, so it is up to you to plan for their protection before a disaster strikes.

There is also a higher risk of spreading communicable diseases like cholera. Depending on the extent of the damage, diseases can easily spread through a displaced community. This is a natural result of a breakdown of hygiene and a lack of supply of potable water to keep the immediate environment clear of contaminants. The ability to wash hands regularly may be limited, and without a solid medical infrastructure, vaccinations may not be readily available. By factoring in all of these possibilities and preparing for them ahead of time, you can protect your family from the onslaught of unexpected health issues that may quickly crop up. By asking yourself, what potential hazards and risks are you most likely to be exposed to in your area and preparing for them ahead of time, you can prevent many of these health conditions from having a major effect on the lives of those in your care.

How to Prepare for Small Children and the Elderly

Your plan becomes a little more complicated when you have to make arrangements for those who are unable to care for themselves. When it comes to family members, not all can follow through on what needs to be done. They may not be able to understand what's happening around them and if they have been historically dependent on you, then that need will most likely increase in the wake of a disaster.

Children, especially the younger ones, lack the maturity to understand catastrophic events that are unfolding around them. You will need to plan for their specific needs in these real world events and help them to cope with the chaos that follows. Needs you will have to address are sheltering, monitoring, evacuation, and training.

This presents a unique set of circumstances that must be dealt with in all areas of a child's life from the neonatal all the way up to the teenage years. To meet these needs, as parents and guardians you must consider their unique circumstances that must be met in getting adequate supplies and care. These include:

- Sleeping needs (cribs, bedding, and clothing)

- Nutritional needs (bottles, safety plates, and child safety utensils, etc.)

- Sanitary needs (diapers, creams, ointments, etc.)

- And medical supplies.

Most small babies are on formulas that may not be readily available after a disaster so it is wise to find a suitable alternative that can be kept free from contamination to use. Instead of the formula, can your baby get by on regular dairy milk or a soy product? Find something that won't trigger digestive problems for them.

When it comes to planning an evacuation, how well will your child be able to keep up with you if you have to move quickly? If they can't, how will you transport them? What type of shelter will you have to be in and how can you help your child to adapt to these new conditions.

You also have to think about the chain of custody. After a disaster, someone will have to be responsible for keeping a watchful eye on these little ones. If you have older children in your family, you could temporarily leave them in charge of a responsible sibling or find a way to manage it yourself.

The same considerations are also needed for the elderly. In any society, these are the individuals who are most likely to get lost or left behind so careful planning for them will not only give your family true peace of mind in a tumultuous time, but it will also ease much of the tension that many people experience after a devastating event has occurred.

Evacuation Plans

After a disaster, you may find that your home is no longer safe for you to stay in. In some cases, the home may still remain intact, but the threat of additional threats to the community may be imminent, and you may be forced to evacuate.

If an entire city or neighborhood has to vacate an area in a short period of time, it can be greatly beneficial to have a plan in place long beforehand. Look around your community to find if any emergency strategies can be put in place to help with the evacuation process.

This strategy will change depending on your particular location. To start creating an evacuation plan, contact your local government agencies to find out if they have any specific evacuation zones for your community. These are often determined based on the type of disaster that may happen in your area and the safest locations to escape to.

For example, someone in a region prone to flooding may be told to flee to higher ground in the case of a rising river. Those who may be faced with a hurricane may have hurricane-safe facilities to go to or may plan to block certain highways if one is approaching.

It is important to locate the nearest approved shelter if evacuations are necessary. This information may not be easy to obtain immediately after something happens and you could lose precious time searching for a safe place to go in the ensuing chaos.

If you have pets, you need to make arrangements for them as well. Many shelters do not have room to accommodate animals along with people. This is not only wise from the perspective of space but also in consideration for the health and safety of the masses. In most situations, people and animals are sheltered separately.

Another thing to consider when developing an evacuation plan is your own mobility. If you are unable to drive or move yourself to a safe location, enlist the aid of someone nearby who will be responsible enough to get you where you need to be. Think about those with wheelchairs, using canes, or in some other way unable to move on their own power.

Look around your immediate community. If you don't have family members close by you can rely on, find some outside assistance that you can expect to come to your aid in the moments immediately after a disaster. Talk to them and make some sort of arrangement to ensure that everyone in your household will reach their designated shelter as quickly and as efficiently as possible.

Once your plan is in place, take it one step further and practice it. Remember those days years ago during the Cold War, when there was a threat of nuclear bombing on the United States? Children were repeatedly drilled over the course of many years to take cover under a desk or some sturdy structure to protect themselves. A teacher needed only to utter one word, "drop!" and students instantly scrambled into action.

We need to have that same mental state when preparing for a disaster with our family. It is not enough to practice it once or twice, but it should become a part of your regular routine. That way, what needs to be done will become so ingrained in the minds of everyone that they will respond to the event without the need to overthink the steps. Your whole family will spring into action and get to safety without the anxiety and fears of those who were not adequately prepared.

Prepare Your Home

Finally, you need to turn your attention to the safety of your home. When a disaster strikes, things get moved around. Furniture that is not secured could topple over and cause injuries, gas and power lines can pose a real threat to occupants, and normal passageways can become blocked.

Preparing your home is more than just carving out a way to the outside. It's securing it in such a way as to not create an additional hazard for the rest of your family.

Those responsible should know where the power boxes are and how to turn off the utilities if they become compromised. Secure areas so that you can you always have a means of escape. Know all the exits in your building in case one is blocked your family knows another way to the outside.

Any chemicals or other types of toxins should be secured to prevent leakage into the environment and set up a rendezvous place for you all to meet if something were to happen. It could be a place nearby or someplace outside of your immediate community.

It helps to plan all of these things together as a family and to rehearse it regularly so that when a disaster does happen, you will know exactly what needs to be done to ensure the safety of your household.

CHAPTER 3

HOW TO PREPARE FOR A TORNADO

In the previous chapter, we discussed what you need to do to prepare for a disaster. The instructions given are not very specific as it was information that everyone household should b considering. However, when you are preparing for something like a tornado or a hurricane you can be even better prepared because you know exactly what to prepare for.

Since tornadoes are known to strike suddenly and no one knows exactly where they will hit it is extremely important to prepare for them ahead of time. Monster tornadoes rip through cities with reckless abandon and not knowing exactly where they will touch down could leave you completely vulnerable if you're not prepared.

On May 22, 2011, the tornado that struck Joplin, Missouri left close to 160 people dead in its wake and thousands injured. With winds packing speeds of over 200 mph, it lasted no more than 22 minutes on the ground, but for miles around, homes were quickly turned into rubble and businesses were literally wiped off the face of the earth. It was one of the worst recorded storms in US history.

With such destruction happening in a short amount of time you are most vulnerable if you aren't prepared. Proper preparation allows you to act quickly as you may only have seconds to get your family to safety.

Know Your Risk

If you live in an area prone to tornadoes you need to be diligent in keeping abreast of warnings and know exactly what to do.

A tornado is a fast moving column of air that is generated in a thunderstorm. The speed at which a tornado move makes it almost impossible to outrun, so it is necessary that you have a secure shelter close by. While there may be a tornado season, they can strike at any time of the year. They are most common, however, in the spring and summer months.

Tornado Warnings

If you live in an area that is susceptible to these destructive forces you need to know what reports actually mean. They can tell you the extent to which you are at risk for a tornado to touch down in your area.

Tornado Watch: When a report says that your area is on a tornado watch it means that a condition for a tornado to develop is possible. If you are not already, it is important to put yourself in a location where you are close enough to a shelter or a building strong enough to withstand the pressures of a tornado if they should develop.

Keep your eyes on the sky for signs of a funnel cloud forming and stay tuned to the NOAA Weather reports or the local news broadcasts.

Tornado Warning: This is a more serious threat as it tells you that a tornado has already been sighted in your area. If you hear this report, you should immediately seek shelter and remain there until you hear an announcement of an all clear.

If your evacuation plan and Bug Out Bag are all ready, you should do this immediately. If your family members are separated, they will know exactly how to get to safety themselves, and after the danger has passed, you can regroup and meet at your predetermined rendezvous point.

What to do During a Tornado

The majority of the injuries sustained in a tornado happen when people are outside of safe shelters. People are struck by flying debris or are picked up and swept away themselves.

If you are away from home (school, hospital, office building, or shopping center) ask for the safest place to hunker down until the danger passes.

- Get to safety immediately. In a tornado, it is best to seek refuge below ground in a basement, cellar, or storage bunker. If there is no underground room to go to, take shelter in the center of the building. The idea is to put as many walls as you can between you and the encroaching storm.

- Once inside, find something sturdy to take cover under. This could be a table or a desk. Look for something that cannot be easily broken.

- Cover yourself with blankets, heavy coats, or pillows to cushion your body from falling debris.

- Use your arms to protect your head and neck from injury.

- If you live in a high-rise building, seek refuge in a small interior hallway or make your way down to the lowest floor possible.

- Keep your windows closed

- Wait it out

For those who live in a lighter weight, manufactured homes, it is best to get outside and find a sturdier structure to wait it out. These types of buildings are usually the first to succumb to the incredible forces of a tornado. Look for a local shelter designated in your community.

If you are outside when a tornado is approaching:

- Look for the strongest building you can find and take shelter there.

- If there is no building around, get into your car, buckle in and try to drive to the closest safe building you can find.

- If your car is struck by flying debris and can no longer drive, pull off the road and park, cover your head and neck with your arms and hide under a blanket or other heavy material for protection.

What Not to do

- Do not take cover under a bridge or an overpass. It is better to be in an open space that is low and flat.

- If you see a tornado, do not try to outrun it, especially in urban or crowded communities.

There is very little you can do when a tornado is bearing down on you, but your primary concern during one is to protect yourself from falling debris. This is the number one cause of fatalities and injuries when a tornado strikes.

What to do After a Tornado

Once a tornado has passed, there is much to do. While imminent danger from flying debris may be over you are still very vulnerable, and you need to know what to do.

- If you are trapped, avoid making any sudden movements. Debris above you may shift and cause a collapse that could rain down on you. To get attention tap on a wall or pipe with something hard. If your Bug Out Bag is equipped with a whistle, you can use that to signal to rescuers where to find you.

- Listen for updates and reports giving you instructions on what to do

- Check-in with your family and friends. If you have cell service, use text messaging and social media rather than calling.

- Examine your property for downed power lines or debris that could cause a hazard

- Do not go into damaged buildings until they have been declared safe by local authorities.

- If you volunteer for post-disaster clean up make sure you wear protective clothing and use extreme caution. Wear long-sleeved shirts, long pants, gloves, and thick-soled shoes.

- Take pictures of your damaged property

- Secure any damaged part of your house against further damage. Seal openings with tarp or plywood, cover holes in the roof and remove any debris that could pose a threat.

- If you are without power, use flashlights or lanterns rather than candles. This prevents the risk of fires breaking out and causing even more devastation.

Even if you are not in an area susceptible to tornadoes, it pays to be aware of these conditions. Windstorms can occur almost anywhere in the country creating a major threat to people and property everywhere. Do not rely on the security that your building is up to governmental codes. Take every precaution you can to secure a safe haven for you and your family.

CHAPTER 4

HOW TO PREPARE FOR
A HURRICANE

Hurricanes can also be very devastating when they strike. These massive storms usually strike hard on coastal regions. They form over the water and build up strength as the move towards land. Protecting yourself from a hurricane involves protection against more than one element striking at the same time. You have to brace yourself against high winds, heavy rainfall, storm surges, and flooding both along the coast and even further inland when necessary. You also need to ward against rip currents and tornadoes that may be generated by a hurricane.

While there is always the potential of a hurricane developing in any coastal region, they are most likely to make landfall in warmer climate regions like along the Atlantic Coast and the Gulf of Mexico. They have been known to reach as far as 100 miles inland and are a constant threat to those who live in the islands of Puerto Rico, Hawaii, the Pacific Southwest, and the Virgin Islands.

Hurricane season usually starts in June and runs through late November but peak season ranges from mid-August to late October. If you live near the Pacific coast, the season begins earlier in May and continues until November.

What to do Before a Hurricane

Even though you may have a few days warning before a hurricane makes landfall, it is a smart move to prepare ahead of time. Generally, when hurricane reports begin, it is not known exactly where its forces will strike. As the storm moves closer to land where it will hit becomes clearer, but if you wait for that, you might find yourselves trapped in a situation where you will have to ride it out. The best course of action:

- Become familiar with safe shelters to seek protection from the storm. If you have been ordered to evacuate, make sure you have a clear and safe route out of the area at risk.

- Get your *Bug Out Bag* and pack and leave as soon as possible.

- If you are not required to evacuate you need to secure your home and make sure you have all the supplies you need to last you a few days. This includes alternative energy and communication sources if you lose these services for a few days.

- Remember, even if you are not expected to evacuate, after the storm you may find yourself trapped due to flooding and damage in surrounding areas.

- Follow your family escape plan.

How to Prepare Your Home

Powerful hurricane force winds are strong enough to uproot trees and lay buildings down flat. Even before you realize that a hurricane is approaching take these steps to secure the safety of your home.

- Trim or remove any trees or branches that may be damaged on your property. These can easily break off in the storm and become projectiles that can cause severe damage to your property.

- Check your rain gutters and downspouts to make sure they are clear of any debris that could clog them up causing a water backup that could damage your property.

- Make sure your roof is secure by reinforcing it. You also want to do the same by retrofitting the windows and doors of your property too.

- Obtain a portable generator for back up power in case you need it.

- Build a safe room as a shelter. These rooms are designed to withstand the forces of a high wind and are often found in locations where residents have to deal with frequent hurricanes.

Know the Warnings

A hurricane watch is a warning that conditions are possible and a hurricane can occur within the next 48 hours. When you hear a hurricane warning, you should never wait for a definitive occurrence but start getting ready immediately.

- Know your evacuation route and be prepared to leave

- Collect your Bug Out Ba and make sure everything is ready to go

- Meet with your family members about what to do if you get separated

- Make arrangements for anyone with disabilities or to help others in your family that may need it.

A hurricane warning means that conditions are right for a hurricane to strike within the next 36 hours.

- Follow evacuation orders given by the local authorities

- Set up communication with all family members both inside and outside the immediate community

- Keep close tabs on the hurricane timeline and make sure all your plans are in place.

- Evacuate as soon as possible if asked to do so

- When the hurricane is 6 hours away

- Make sure your TV/radio or website is on and giving regular updates on the hurricane's progress

- If you're not evacuating, make sure you're stocked up for a long-term housebound situation

- Let others outside the affected area know where you will be

- Close your storm shutters and cover the windows to prevent flying debris from getting into your home.

- Turn up the refrigerator and freezer to the highest setting and start restricting access to maintain the cold temperature even if the power goes out.

- Charge up your cell phones and any batteries you may need

- Start bringing in any loose or lightweight objects inside to secure them. Patio furniture, garbage containers, and other things outside your home should be stored safely away.

- Make sure your car is gassed up and ready to go. Stock it with all of your emergency supplies so you can flee at a moment's notice.

What to do After a Hurricane

There is little to do during a hurricane except wait it out, but once it is over, you still need to exercise caution.

- Don't venture outside until after you've heard reports that the storm has passed

- Immediately check in with family and friends to let them know you're safe.

- If you've evacuated, wait for the authorities to tell you it's safe to go back to your neighborhood.

- Keep a careful eye on the debris and possible downed power lines.

- Stay away from flooded roads and pathways. It only takes a few inches of water to sweep you away. It could also be electrically charged from downed power lines.

- Take pictures of any damage to your property.

- Start cleaning up and securing areas where damage could create a potential risk to life and limb.

- Restock your Bug Out Bag so it is ready for the next disaster that might strike.

CHAPTER 5

WHAT TO DO WHEN AN EARTHQUAKE STRIKES

Unlike other disastrous situations, earthquakes strike without warning. There are usually no signs in the weather or the environment that can tell you that an earthquake is imminent. The sudden shaking of the ground beneath you can trigger a wide range of frightful experiences as the earth breaks free from its holds releasing strains that may have built up over thousands of years.

Generally, earthquakes start with a mild shaking that gradually builds up in intensity over the next few seconds. They can be very light feeling like a general rolling or rocking sensation, but they can quickly become extremely violent.

Stronger earthquakes are often followed by smaller aftershocks, which can continue at unexpected intervals and last for months afterward.

Earthquakes can also trigger other disastrous events that could be equally, if not more devastating like tsunamis, the collapsing of buildings, bridges, roads, and dams. In certain situations, they could also trigger landslides, avalanches, and widespread fire.

Considering that you only have a matter of seconds to respond to an earthquake, it is more important than ever to be prepared before one strikes. The decision could make the difference between life and death for your entire family.

Who is at Risk?

It may come as a surprise to know that the entire United States is at risk for some type of earthquake. However, those at higher risk are those in already identified highly active seismic zones. These include those areas around the San Andreas Fault in California, the Oregon Cascadia Subjunction Zone, and the states of Washington and Alaska.

Other areas that are considered high risk are the New Madrid Fault Zone that passes through Missouri, Arkansas, Tennessee, and Kentucky and the Mid-Atlantic region on the east coast, as well as South Carolina and New England states.

What to do Before an Earthquake

Your best bet for protection is to have a plan in place before an earthquake strikes.

- Secure your home by making sure items in cabinets and on shelves cannot easily fall down. This includes bolting bookshelves, mirrors, and large appliances in place. Light fixtures should be firmly in place, computers, televisions, hot water heaters, etc. should be secured as well.

- Beds and furniture where people tend to relax and sleep should be placed away from windows and away from anything that might fall down on them.

- Rehearse how to take cover quickly with your family by preparing drop and cover drills with them.

- Show children how to dive under a table or desk and cover their head and neck with their arms.

- If no safe place is nearby, teach them how to crawl to a safer location and not to try to stand and walk. When the ground is shaking it is better to stay low to avoid the risk of injury.

- Before an earthquake happens is the time to prepare. Because they come on so suddenly, there is no time to think when it happens. With only seconds available for you to find cover, your response time must become second nature to you, and that requires lots and lots of practice.

What to do During an Earthquake

If you are inside:

- When the earth is moving, you should have only one thing on your mind. How to protect yourself from falling debris. As soon as you feel movement in the earth, drop down on your hands and knees and cover your head and neck with your arms.

- If you're at risk from falling objects, try to move to a safer area. Take cover under a desk or a table for the best protection.

- Move away from windows or large objects that might fall on you.

- Try to find an interior hallway or wall and get as close to it as possible.

- Find something strong and stable and hug it tightly until the shaking stops.

- Once you find cover, move as little as possible until the shaking comes to a complete stop.

- Do not attempt to run outside during an earthquake

- Try to stay away from doorways as you might get hit with flying debris

If you are in bed:

- Stay there and cover your head and neck with a pillow

- Do not try to run for safety. Objects are difficult to see at night, and you could put yourself in more danger by running in the darkness.

- If you are outside:

- Try to move as far away from buildings as possible

- Avoid streetlights, power lines, and other potential hazards that may come down.

If you are in a moving vehicle:

- It is almost impossible to drive during an earthquake.

- Stop as quickly as it is safe to do so and remain inside your vehicle

- Stay away from buildings, trees, utility wires, bridges, overpasses, etc.

What to do After an Earthquake

It is important to remember that once the shaking stops, the danger is not over. You may come out from your cover but do so cautiously.

- Survey the area around you to make sure it is safe.

- If your immediate area appears safe, try to secure a safe passage to the outside.

- Leave only when you have a pathway to a clear area of safety away from falling debris.

- If you are trapped inside, keep your movements slow and minimal.

- Use a cell phone and text for help

- Tap on a wall or pipe to alert rescuers where you are

- Assess your injuries on yourself and those around you.

- If you are able, offer assistance when needed.

- If you are near the coast, move inland or up to higher ground as quickly as possible: the threat of tsunamis and liquefaction could put you in more jeopardy.

- Take extra care when doing post-earthquake cleanup – do not attempt to move heavy pieces of debris on your own, get help.

- Wear proper attire.

- Always be alert for safe places to go when aftershocks occur – remember, it's not over until it's over.

CHAPTER 6

WHAT TO DO IN AN AVALANCHE

If you are in regions where there is lots of snow, there is usually a risk of avalanches. Like earthquakes, these can happen with little or no warning with thousands of tons of snow, ice, and any debris it can carry along with it racing downhill at incredible speeds.

Every year, skiers, and other winter enthusiasts find themselves right in the path of an avalanche with only seconds to take action. It is imperative that you know what to do as soon as you realize you're in danger.

What to do Before an Avalanche

Since there is no way of knowing exactly when and

where an avalanche will happen your safety depends on how well you have observed your environment and prepared beforehand.

- Make sure you're wearing a rescue beacon that can help search and rescue to find you

- Learn how to use any equipment used in snow rescues

- Always be aware of your surroundings and know the risk of avalanches in your location

- Watch out for any area that has a fresh accumulation of snow (especially wind-driven snow) as they are the most vulnerable

- Stay away from steep slopes located in areas with lots of shade or that are near a ridge or cliff

- Never go out without a partner so both of you can watch for signs of a potential avalanche

- Avoid drifting into any terrain without proper equipment. Always carry a probe to help with searching for buried survivors, a beacon, and a shovel and learn how to use them properly

- Wear an avalanche airbag. These can keep you on top of the slide so you won't get buried deep under the snow, increasing your odds of survival.

- Wear a helmet to avoid getting struck in the head by any other objects that may be swept away by the avalanche.

What You Can Do If You're Caught in an Avalanche

- If you're caught in a slide, try to roll off and grab onto a tree.

- Hug it until the slide passes

- If unable to break away, swim for the surface as soon as you can

- If not, try not to move and wait for rescue

Rescue Efforts

- Carry a small shovel in the event your partner is buried, you can begin to dig them out as soon as it is safe

- Do not begin to dig until you have evaluated the surroundings to avoid triggering a second avalanche

In an avalanche, you not only have the risk of injury from being swept away by the fast-moving snow but you also have the risk of hyperthermia if you're buried alive. If caught in the flow your chances of survival lie in how quickly rescue workers can find you and how well you're prepared. Reports show that victims found within 15 minutes have the greater chance of survival. After that, the odds drop drastically. Only 20% of victims can survive for 45 minutes or more after being buried in the snow.

CHAPTER 7

WHAT TO DO IN A FLOOD

In a flood, water rises quickly and can easily overtake people, objects, and homes washing them away in a matter of seconds. It doesn't take a lot of water to create a dangerous situation that can put lives at risk. These dangerous waters can appear in any location without warning.

Floods are not always the result of heavy rainfall or melting snowcaps, they could be the result of nearby storms, storm surges, an overflow of waterways, or the blocking of wastewater systems. While some floods happen slowly giving you time to react flash floods usually develop rapidly with little or no warning.

Basic Safety Precautions

- Whenever you see a pool of water in a location where it is usually dry, do not try to cross it. Without knowing what's in it or how deep it is you could easily be injured or carried away.

- Do not cross bridges where there is fast moving water flowing underneath it. These waters can erode the foundation around the footing causing the bridge to become unstable.

- Remember only a few inches of water can knock you down and sweep you away, and only a foot of water can move a vehicle

- If there is any chance of flood, move to higher ground.

- If you can't drive to higher ground, it is better to abandon your car and move on foot.

- If your vehicle is caught in a flood, do not attempt to leave the car and get into the moving water

- Do not camp or linger too close to streams, rivers, or creeks when there has been a lot of rain.

Know the Warning Signs

A flood watch is when the conditions are right for a flood, and the potential is high:

- If you hear a report of a flood watch, stay tuned to any broadcasts and emergency instructions

- Already know where you will go and your means of getting to higher ground

- Get your Bug Out Bag ready and make sure everything is prepared.

- Secure your home

  - Bring in anything that could be washed away and secure valuables on the highest level possible in your home

  - Disconnect all electrical appliances

o   Turn off the gas and electricity to the house from the main switch

A flood warning means that a flood is actually happening or will definitely happen soon.

- Take immediate action

- Move to higher ground and stay there until you get an all clear

- Evacuate if instructed to do so

- Do not walk or drive through any flood waters

What to do After the Flood

- Only return home when you've received an all clear from the authorities

- Watch out for debris that may still be buried underwater

- Don't assume any place is safe, flood waters can erode roads, paths, and walkways making them unstable

- Do not cross standing water. It could be electrically charged from downed power lines or underground cables

- Photograph any damage to your property

CHAPTER 8

WHAT TO DO IN AN ACTIVE SHOOTER SITUATION

Aside from the natural disasters that can strip us of our quality of life, there are also man-made disasters that we are now forced to have to cope with. With increasing frequency, we are hearing reports of shootings in schools, theaters, workplaces, and even in places of worship. All of this increases our threat assessment and puts us in jeopardy no matter where we are.

Unlike natural disasters that have been around for thousands of years, active shooting situations are something that is relatively new to our society, and as a result, few people know how to react or respond in such situations.

While the risk of finding yourself in this type of situation is still relatively low compared to other disasters, many disaster preparedness experts believe the trend will continue and therefore encourage everyone to think about the possibility and know ahead of time what they should do in such a situation.

They recommend the three-step approach:

- Run

- Hide

- Fight

Unfortunately, since this event could happen just about any place and at any time, it is unlikely that you will find a standard set of rules to help you prepare. Most of the actions you must take require quick mental thinking to protect yourself. Still, there are some simple guidelines that can help you to find safety in the event you're caught in such a situation.

An active shooter situation is a precarious one at best and the more knowledge you have about the circumstances, the safer you could be so before finding yourself in an event, it pays to learn as much as you can about these highly volatile tragedies.

What to do Before an Active Shooter Situation

Since there are no clear signs that an active shooter is in your midst, you need to be very aware of your surroundings no matter where you go.

- Always keep your eyes open for the nearest exit, especially when you're in a crowded environment

- If you notice something that doesn't seem right – report it to the authorities immediately.

- Take extra care if you are in a new and unfamiliar location

- Only use exits when you are sure that they will not take you directly into the path of the gunman

- Sign up for an active shooter training course

What to do During an Active Shooter Situation

If possible, escape

- Your primary concern is safety. If you find there is an active shooter in your midst, leave your belongings and escape as fast as you can

- Help others to escape if possible

- Shout a warning to anyone who may be heading in the direction of the shooter

- When you reach safety, call for emergency assistance

- If you were able to get a good look at the shooter, provide a description including the clothes he was wearing, the location you last saw him, and the kind of weapons he was carrying.

If escape is not possible, hide

- Find a place to hide that is out of the shooter's range of sight and cannot be penetrated by the shooter's weapons

- Remain very quiet

- Put all electronic devices on silent or turn them off completely

- Lock and block all doors, close any blinds or windows and turn off lights

- Avoid hiding with groups of people – it's better to hide separately so you won't be so easy to find

- If possible, send a silent message to authorities – use text or social media, post a sign in a window or find another way to let them know you need help

- Stay in place until the rescuers arrive and give you the all clear

- If you come face to face with the shooter

- Do not hesitate, be as aggressive as possible

- Call for others to help in creating an ambush

- Use whatever you can as a weapon – chairs, books, fire extinguishers, pencils, knives, scissors (you are fighting for your life)

- Throw items to distract his attention and prevent him from shooting at you

- If you have a chance to get away, run in a zigzag pattern so he can't get a good aim or run from cover to cover

- DO NOT pull the fire alarm. It can add to the chaos and send others right into the shooter's path

- As you escape, yell "gun!" or "shooter!" so others are warned

After you get the all clear, there will still be a lot of chaos and confusion with both the others in the situation and law enforcement. To avoid being a suspect yourself, it is best to follow these basic guidelines.

- Walk out with your hands empty but visible

- Expect that officers may use non-lethal weapons in these situations (pepper spray or tear gas) especially if they have not identified the shooter yet.

- Follow their directions as they give commands to you

- If they push you down forcibly or treat you roughly, understand it is for your protection

- Take care of yourself first before attempting to help others who may have been injured

- Help others to safety if you can

- If people are wounded, turn them over on their side

- If they are unconscious, find a way to keep them warm

- Seek counseling from a professional to help you cope with the long-term psychological effects like PTSD

When an active gunman is on the premise, panic is usually their best weapon. It causes people to run out into the open making themselves an easy target. The more you prepare mentally ahead of time, the less likely you will become one of those victims, and you can get yourself to safety.

CHAPTER 9

WHAT TO DO IN
A TERRORIST ATTACK

Terrorist attacks come in all forms. They could be bombs going off in unexpected places, toxic gases released in public locations, they could be hijacked planes, or vehicles plowing through a crowd of people.

It is difficult to have a plan when you don't know the form or shape of the enemy, but some basic and simple guidelines can help you to stay safe. While in some situations there are no means of escape, it is still important to know what you can do to help yourself if at all possible.

- Run

- Hide

- Tell

It is important to understand that the advice given here is relatively new and has only been released officially within the past year. These suggestions may be updated from time to time to keep up with this growing trend in public dangers.

Run

If you find yourself in a situation where you can get out quickly, law enforcement officials recommend that you do so as quickly as you can. In cases where there are one or more gunmen, this is the best course of action. If you are located in a high-rise building, and ground floor exit is not possible, run to the rooftop where you can signal for help. Try to put as much distance between you and the gunman as possible.

Hide

Look for some type of shelter where you can hide. Look for places to conceal yourself where you can lock yourself in and create a barricade. A bathroom, a closet, or someplace where the gunman will have to work to get at you are usually the best option.

Fight

If nothing else and you have no options to run or hide, be ready to fight.

What to do if it is a Bomb Attack

In the case of a bomb attack, the dangers are usually present after the bomb explodes.

- If at all possible, leave the area as quickly as you can

- Help those you can to get out to safety

- Stay far away from any damaged buildings

- Watch out for falling debris or glass

If you can't get out:

- Find a sturdy place to take cover

- Stay away from gas lines or power lines

- When moving through the building do not take the elevator.

- Call for help – let authorities know your location, where you last saw the suspects, and give any other descriptions that can help them

- Inform first responders of any casualties, injuries, or any information that can help them to navigate the building better

- If you are injured, seek medical attention as soon as possible

- Be patient – if your injuries are not serious, you may have to wait a while to get the treatment you need.

If you are traveling:

- Learn high traffic areas in your new location and avoid them. They can become a terrorist target

- Only visit locations that have good security measures in place

- Learn your surroundings, so you don't get lost in the chaos

- Avoid any locations where large masses of people are demonstrating

- Learn the contact numbers of emergency services

- Find the location of your embassy

- Have a rendezvous point for anyone traveling with you

- Create an evacuation plan as soon as you arrive

- Buy travel insurance

What to do After a Terrorist Attack

Keep in mind that a terrorist's goal is to create chaos and panic. Their attacks are intended to be extremely stressful so make sure you keep your head.

- As soon as you can, contact your embassy to let them know your location. If you are alright, and to request assistance

- Always carry something that can soothe your nerves. Some people carry a family photo, their favorite music, a religious icon, or another cherished possession

- Get medical treatment as soon as possible if needed.

Offer Medical Assistance

If you are not injured, offer help to those who are.

- If you find someone who is unconscious but is still breathing – check to make sure they have no other injuries. If not, turn them over on their side and wait for assistance

- If they are not breathing, administer CPR as soon as possible

- If they are bleeding – apply pressure to the wound to stop the bleeding

Terrorist attacks are meant to disrupt the infrastructure and the workings of the point of attack. By offering assistance and resisting the urge to panic you defeat the purpose of the terrorist and disrupt their actions instead.

CONCLUSION

Thank for making it through to the end of this book, let's hope it was informative and able to provide you with all of the tools you need to achieve your goals whatever they may be.

It doesn't matter who we are, where we live, or what we know, disasters are an equal opportunity tragedy. Whether you're in California preparing for the Big One or you're in Florida gearing up for the next hurricane. Very few people go through life without having to face imminent danger at some point.

It makes perfect sense then that we arm ourselves and are proactive when it comes to protecting our lives and the lives of those around us. Through the pages of this book, we have covered many details that can help us to know what is coming, and how to be prepared for it.

This book is a true gift. It teaches you not only how to help yourselves but extend a helping hand to those around you. By following the guidelines we've set up in this book, you will be able to face each situation, no matter how catastrophic, with confidence that you have done all you can do. Whether you have a plan for before, during, and after you can be sure that you have geared up for the worst of it and are prepared to go the distance.

Finally, if you found this book useful in any way, a review on Amazon is always appreciated!